Keep Yourself Healthy

God's Principles of Good Health

Neil G. Bauman, Th.D., Ph.D.

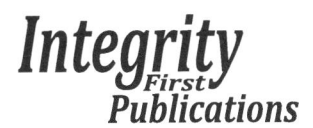

Integrity First Publications

Stewartstown, PA   http://www.IntegrityFirstPublications.com

Keep Yourself Healthy
God's Principles of Good Health

Third Edition

Another **Integrity First** book in the series:

Get More (Much More) Out of Your Bible

Copyright 1994, 2005, 2011 by Neil G. Bauman

ISBN 978-1-935939-15-3

All rights reserved. No part of this publication may be reproduced or transmitted in any form or by any means, electronic or mechanical, including photocopying, recording or any other information storage and retrieval system without permission in writing from the publisher, except by a reviewer who may quote brief passages in a review.

Cover photo: Great Blue Heron, photographed by Neil Bauman.

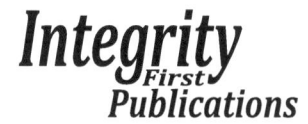

Integrity First Publications

49 Piston Court,
Stewartstown, PA 17363-8322
Phone: (717) 993-8555
FAX: (717) 993-6661
Email: info@IntegrityFirstPublications.com
Website: http://www.IntegrityFirstPublications.com

Printed in the United States of America

Contents

About the Author 5

Preface 7

1. God Wants Us to Be Healthy! 9

2. God's Public Health Laws Examined 11
    Quarantine..11
    Sanitation 13
    Personal Cleanliness......................................14

3. Law and Grace: Not, Law or Grace 17

4. God's Dietary Laws..19
    God's Answer to Fat..20
    It's a Bloody Business....................................22
    Fit Flesh for Humans......................................24

5. **Results of Breaking God's Dietary Laws............27**
    Trichinosis 27
    Cancer 31
    Paralytic Shellfish Poisoning..........................33
    Liver Cirrhosis...38

6. **Unclean Animals Aptly Named 41**

7. **But the New Testament Says............................45**

Literature Cited 55

Bible-Based Books by the Same Author 59

About the Author

Neil Bauman is an evangelical, Bible-believing Christian. He grew up under the tutelage of Dr. Herbert Robinson, his first pastor and mentor. Dr. Robinson taught him how to delve deeply into the Word of God and discover the many truths hidden below the surface—things that most people miss in their cursory reading of the Bible. In addition to researching the deeper truths in the Word of God, Dr. Neil delights in teaching and sharing what he has learned with others.

He earned two doctorates from the former Northgate Graduate School—a Doctor of Philosophy (1981) and a Doctor of Theology (1986).

Dr. Neil began following God's health laws as a teenager. He has been interested in good health ever since. For the past 50 plus years he has proved the wisdom of following God's dietary laws.

Dr. Neil's other passion is helping people successfully live with their hearing losses. He is a

Keep Yourself Healthy

recognized authority in this field, having written 11 books and more than 600 articles related to hearing loss.

    You can reach Dr. Neil at:

Neil Bauman, Ph.D.
49 Piston Court
Stewartstown, PA 17363
Phone: (717) 993-8555
FAX: (717) 993-6661
Email: neil@hearinglosshelp.com
Website: http://www.hearinglosshelp.com
Website: http://www.integrityfirstpublications.com

Preface

God loves us and wants us to be healthy! Since God designed us and made us, He knows what makes us "tick". Likewise, He also knows what harms our health. That is why He put His rules for good health in His Word to us, the Bible.

Unfortunately, far too many people are sick because they either don't know or ignore God's instructions for good health.

Keep Yourself Healthy only deals with one specific aspect of good health, namely, God's biblical health rules. Furthermore, it is not an exhaustive treatment on this subject. Rather, it is a beginner's book, guiding those interested in good health into a fuller understanding of God's health rules.

At the same time, do not ignore the many other essential aspects of good health that are not studied here. These include such things as proper nutrition, exercise, rest, relaxation, sexual purity and good mental, emotional and spiritual health. Fortunately, there are many excellent books available on these subjects.

All biblical quotations are from the New King James version of the Bible unless otherwise noted.

Chapter 1

God Wants Us to Be Healthy

God wants us to be healthy! He is the loving God who heals all our diseases (Psalms 103:3). The disciple John wrote, "Beloved, I pray that you may prosper in all things and be in **health**" (III John 2). King Solomon in his wisdom stated, "My son, give attention to my words; ... for they [God's words] are **life** to those who find them, And **health** to all their flesh" (Proverbs 4:20, 22). He also wrote, "**Do not be wise in your own eyes**; Fear the Lord and depart from evil. It will be **health** to your flesh, and strength to your bones" (Proverbs 3:7-8).

Furthermore, God declared, "If you **diligently heed** the voice of the Lord your God and **do what is right** in His sight, give ear to His **commandments** and **keep all His statutes**, I [the Lord] will put **none of the diseases** on you which I have brought on the Egyptians. For **I am the Lord who heals you**" (Exodus 15:26).

Some of us get sick because we are ignorant of God's health laws. In fact, God laments, "My people are destroyed for **lack of knowledge**" (Hosea 4:6). Yet we have no excuse for our Bibles contain this very knowledge we need.

Others of us get sick because we willfully, yes, willfully, reject God's health laws. God declared, "you have **rejected knowledge**" (Hosea 4:6), so we reap the results. God warns us, "the curse without cause does not come" (Proverbs 26:2, NASB). Thus, we have to accept the consequences for our actions. We invite disease and death when we step outside the safety zone of God's Word. We have only ourselves to blame if we then get sick.

God gives us two choices. Either we obey His commandments, keep His statutes and be healthy, or else disobey His laws, ignore His statutes and risk getting sick or even dying.

Chapter 2

God's Public Health Laws Examined

God has much to say about health. Remember, He wants us to be healthy. The Bible contains His laws on public health. Let's consider a few of them.

Quarantine

Did you know that for over 1,000 years, from about A.D. 400 until A.D. 1500,[1] leprosy was a dreaded killer of millions of people in Europe?[2] You knew about the Black Plague, of course, but leprosy? In fact, leprosy was "the greatest disease of medieval Christendom."[3]

Dr. George Rosen wrote of how leprosy threw its terrorizing shadow over the daily life of medieval humanity. In fact, the fear of all other diseases was not equal to the terror spread by leprosy. Neither the Black Death in the fourteenth century nor the outbreak of syphilis near the end of the fifteenth century produced such dread and fear.[4]

From its beginning in the fifth century, leprosy quickly spread throughout Europe. There it became a serious social and health problem, particularly among the poor. Its effects intensified and during the thirteenth and fourteenth centuries reached terrifying proportions.[5]

Dr. McMillen, in his excellent book, **None of These Diseases**, describes the ignorance and impotence of the physicians. Some taught that it was caused by eating hot foods, peppers and garlic or else from eating the meat of diseased hogs. Others, obviously more astrologer than doctor, felt that malign conjunctions of the planets were responsible. Of course, all of these suggestions to prevent leprosy were utterly worthless.[6]

So how was the leprosy plague in Europe finally controlled? Surprisingly, the Church took control and turned to the Bible for direction as the physicians had nothing else left to offer.[7] The Church followed God's instructions as found in Leviticus, chapter 13. In this chapter, God meticulously described how to diagnose leprosy. He told what steps to take to prevent its spread. These steps included isolating all infected people, washing or disposing of infected clothes and even houses, and cleansing others who had come in contact with infected persons. Finally, He described the signs of a healed person who then returned to everyday society.

Some have even reported that Leviticus 13 is our first model of sanitary legislation.[8] Yes, God said it first!

In Europe, the Church began to control leprosy when they segregated or quarantined all lepers according to God's law. At the peak of this plague in the fifteenth century, there were at least 19,000 leper houses (sanitariums) in England, France, Germany and Spain alone.[9]

When the European nations saw how using the practical scriptural principles of quarantine brought leprosy under control, they applied this same principle to control the bubonic plague epidemic with equally spectacular results. Their actions saved millions of lives.[10]

Sanitation

Deadly epidemics such as typhoid, cholera and dysentery have occurred and still occur in many places where the people do not follow God's public health rules on sanitation.

What was God's way? "You shall set off a place outside the camp [a latrine or outhouse] and, when you go out to use it, you must carry a spade . . . and dig a hole, have easement, and turn to cover the excrement" (Deuteronomy 23:12-13, Berkeley).

The world's way was decidedly different. Normally the people dumped their excrement into the filthy, unpaved streets. As a result, powerful stenches gripped villages and cities. Myriads of flies bred in this filth and spread such intestinal diseases as typhoid, cholera and dysentery that killed millions.[11]

As late as the Spanish-American War in 1898, almost 2,000 U. S. troops died of disease.[12] Many others got sick but recovered. Again, this was a direct result of disregarding God's sanitary laws.[13]

Think of the enormous waste of human lives. These people could have saved their lives if they had just obeyed God's rules of sanitation.

Personal Cleanliness

Another of God's public health principles to prevent the spread of disease was personal hygiene or cleanliness (See Numbers 19:11-19).

In Vienna, as elsewhere in the world in the 1840's, one out of every six women in maternity wards at good hospitals died soon after childbirth. The doctors of the day put their deaths down to constipation, delayed lactation, fear and poisonous air.[14]

The doctors performed autopsies on these bodies each morning. Without washing their hands, clothes or implements, these doctors then marched into the wards to perform the necessary pelvic exams.

One bright young doctor, Ignaz Semmelweis, observed that the examined women often died. He reasoned that something was being carried from patient to patient. In his ward, he decreed that each doctor must wash his hands before going from the morgue to the patients.

The results were spectacular. From one in six dying, the death toll dropped to only one in eighty-four! Eventually, he had his doctors wash between examining each patient and the death toll again fell dramatically.[15]

Nor are we exempt here in North America. For example, in 1958 a staphylococcus infection caused

Chapter 2: God's Public Health Laws Examined

by improperly washed hands swept through a large hospital in New York state. This alarmed the New York State Department of Health. Because these infections are spread quickly and easily by a person who doesn't wash his hands properly, they quickly took action. In 1960, the Department published a book showing the proper way to wash the hands. This way closely follows the Biblical method given in Numbers 19.[16]

Chapter 2 Endnotes

1. Leprosy, 1979. p. 180.
2. McMillen, 1978. p. 11.
3. Leprosy, 1910. p. 479.
4. McMillen, 1978. p. 11.
5. McMillen, 1978. p. 11.
6. McMillen, 1978. p. 11.
7. McMillen, 1978. p. 11.
8. McMillen, 1978. p. 12.
9. Leprosy, 1910. p. 480.
10. McMillen, 1978. p. 12.
11. McMillen, 1978. p. 13.
12. Spanish-American War, 1910. p. 598
13. Josephson, 1976. p. 162.
14. McMillen, 1978. p. 13.
15. McMillen, 1978. pp. 13-14.
16. McMillen, 1978. p. 16.

Chapter 3

Law and Grace: Not, Law or Grace

These foregoing examples came from the public health laws quoted from three often-ignored Old Testament books: Leviticus, Numbers and Deuteronomy. Why are they so often ignored? Because too many Christians conclude that because we do not live under law, but under grace, we do not have to keep these Old Testament laws.

Before you make the same mistake, notice that each of these illustrations occurred during this present Christian age, the age of grace. Yet multiplied millions of people in Europe died. Over 60 million died in the Black Plague[1] because they broke God's law while living under grace. Notice also, in each of the above cases, the people only overcame these diseases when they finally obeyed these supposedly obsolete Old Testament public health laws.

Jesus' death on the cross did not free us from these Old Testament laws. Jesus' death only freed us from the curse of the law (Galatians 3:13). That is, we don't lose our salvation for breaking one of these laws. However, break one of God's public health laws and you may meet the Lord far sooner than you had ever anticipated!

Actually, you can't break one of God's laws. That's why we call them laws in the first place. You just break yourself on them.

Chapter 3 Endnotes

1   McMillen, 1978. p. 11.

Chapter 4

God's Dietary Laws

Why have we still not learned that **all** of God's dietary laws, like His public health laws, are for **our benefit**? Why don't we realize we must obey them if we want good health? For example, most people (including Christians who should know better) daily break God's dietary laws. Yet God considered these dietary laws so important that He placed them in Leviticus 11:1-47 and repeated them again in Deuteronomy 14:3-21 to be sure we didn't miss them.

Get this straight. God planned that we must eat to live. So also, God planned that we must eat the right foods to be healthy. Eat—live. Don't eat—die. Eat proper foods—live healthy. Eat wrong foods—get sick. Its that simple.

Now let's consider some of God's dietary laws and see their application to our lives.

God's Answer to Fat

Our loving God declared that we are not to eat animal fat, period. "You shall not eat any fat, of ox or sheep or goat. And the fat of an animal that dies naturally, and the fat of what is torn by wild beasts may be used **in any other way**; but **you shall by no means eat it**" (Leviticus 7:23-24).

Animal fats cause trouble in our bodies! We all know how modern medicine has linked eating animal fats to heart disease and clogged arteries. Why didn't we listen to God? After all, He said it first, in 1,453 B. C. to be exact.

Today, heart disease kills millions each year around the world. In 1974, for example, 974,000 people died of heart and circulatory diseases in the United States alone. In the same year over 30 million Americans suffered from major forms of heart and circulatory diseases.[1]

A high fat diet is a major cause of heart disease. Here is how it happens. Our bodies absorb these fats into our blood streams as fatty protein molecules. Our bodies then deposit large amounts of lipids such as blood fats, cholesterol and triglycerides on our artery walls.[2] By and by, we burn off the proteins and fats leaving the cholesterol behind. As the cholesterol piles up, it irritates the artery wall and encourages more such deposits. Eventually, our blood has a hard time squeezing through our narrowed arteries and we end up with high blood pressure. Ultimately, heart attacks or strokes claim us.[3]

The following two examples attest that this was as true in Old Testament times as it is today.

Chapter 4: God's Dietary Laws

The high priest Eli and his two sons, Hophni and Phinehas, were gluttons. In the days when Samuel was still a lad, they had quite a racket going! They definitely didn't follow God's laws.

Here was God's plan for sacrifices. When the people brought a sacrifice to the Lord, they brought it to a priest. The priest cut off the fat and burned it (Leviticus 3:3-5). He then roasted the meat and kept a portion for himself and the other priests.

Eli's two sons weren't having any of that. They ordered their servants to get them raw meat, **fat and all**. If anyone protested that God's law required that they cut the fat off first and roast the meat, they seized the sacrifice by force and took what they wanted (I Samuel 2:15-16).

As a result of disobeying God, Eli and his sons became **fat** (I Samuel 2:29, 4:18). However, God was displeased and judged them. In fulfillment of God's judgment, Eli's two sons died in a battle. When Eli heard this news, he was so overcome with grief that he toppled backwards off his chair. In the process, he broke his neck because he was so heavy (I Samuel 4:17-18). Furthermore, God declared that Eli's descendants would all die in their prime (I Samuel 2:33). Here a line of gluttons seem to have suffered fatal heart attacks because of their obesity and their love of eating fat. Yes, God truly visits the sins of the fathers upon their children (Exodus 34:7).

Coming back to this present century, the Rev. Elmer Josephson tells of visiting a couple who had both suffered strokes. The lady who was grossly overweight was now paralyzed and blind. Upon closer investigation, he discovered that faulty nutrition had caused her serious condition. Although their animal fat intake was dangerously high, she made no attempt to correct it and died soon afterward.

Her husband, although completely paralyzed on one side, was more fortunate. A neighbor helped take care of him. This neighbor understood the importance of proper nutrition and took him off all animal fats. Instead, he was fed fresh vegetables, grains, nuts and fruits.[4]

Several months later Rev. Josephson again visited the man whom he thought would be in bed sick or by then, even dead. Imagine his surprise when he found the formerly paralyzed man outside hoeing his garden. He had made a complete recovery in a relatively short time. He had bent over backward obeying the scriptural injunction to eat no fat and had fully regained his health![5]

Nor is heart disease the only disease we get from eating animal fat. Researchers are just now discovering that there seems to be a link between eating animal fat and certain kinds of cancer such as breast cancer and colorectal cancer.[6]

It's a Bloody Business

Eating blood in any form is forbidden. Had not God explicitly commanded, "Moreover you shall not eat any blood in any of your dwellings, whether of bird or beast" (Leviticus 7:26)?

Eating blood is bad for us because as God says, "the life of the flesh is in the blood" (Leviticus 17:11). This includes the many diseases that we carry around in our bloodstreams. Just imagine the animal equivalent of the AIDS virus to get the picture.

Chapter 4: God's Dietary Laws

Multiply this by the hundreds of different diseases that animals are susceptible to. No wonder that blood is the first part of a butchered animal to putrefy!

Disease does not come without a cause. Mr. J_____'s grandmother was a Swedish Christian. She was afraid of cancer and prayed all her life that she would not die from that dreaded disease. God, however ignored her prayers, and she died of cancer. Why?

We find the answer in her lifestyle. She kept hogs. When the time came to butcher them, she saved their blood to make blood sausage, a real delicacy to her.[7] She did not just disobey God's direct command and eat blood. She went further and compounded her sin by eating pig's blood. Pigs, God had declared, are not fit food for humans. Therefore, He had strictly forbidden people from ever eating them. Thus she signed her own death warrant. What could God do?

Perhaps you say, "I don't eat blood. I can't stand the thought of a blood pudding or blood sausage." Well then, what about all the blood-soaked meat you buy in the supermarket? It certainly wasn't killed according to God's standard, that is, with **all** the blood drained out. Today, blood is deliberately left in the meat to make it weigh more. Thus there are more profits for the butcher. Furthermore, they think blood in the meat makes the meat taste better.[8]

Abstaining from eating blood is so important to our health that God waves a red warning flag in front of our eyes. Notice how He repeats and emphasizes this law again and again.

"Only **be sure that you do not eat the blood**, for the blood is the life; you may not eat the life with the meat. **You shall not eat it**; you shall pour it on

23

the earth like water. **You shall not eat it**, that it may **go well with you** and your children after you, **when you do what is right** in the sight of the Lord" (Deuteronomy 12:23-25).

And again. "This shall be a **perpetual statute** throughout your generations in all your dwellings: **you shall eat neither fat nor blood**" (Leviticus 3:17).

Fit Flesh for Humans

In Leviticus 11 and Deuteronomy 14 God sets out simple rules to determine which animals are good food for humans. God divided all living creatures into four groups:

1. land animals
2. water animals and fish
3. flying animals and birds
4. insects.

To be fit for human food, land animals must meet two criteria. The animal must have a **split hoof and** it must **chew its cud**. Biologists call these animals ungulates. They include cattle, sheep, goats, deer, moose, elk, antelope, gazelles and similar animals (Leviticus 11:3).

Forbidden land animals include pigs, horses, bears, rabbits, camels, animals that have paws—in other words all land animals that aren't ungulates.

Animals and fish that live in the oceans, lakes and rivers also must meet two criteria. They must have both **fins and scales** (Leviticus 11:9). Those fish that are good for food look like the typical fish found in our waters. They include bass, cod, halibut, herring, perch, pike, salmon, sardines, smelt, sole, trout, white fish and many others.

Those marine animals God declares unfit for human food (and thus bad for your health) in this group include all shellfish such as clams, oysters, lobsters, crabs, shrimp and prawns. As well, they include squid, octopus, sharks, sturgeon (and caviar), eels, whales, seals, frogs and snakes.

The birds are more difficult to specify. The Bible only lists those that we are not to eat (Leviticus 11:13-19). All others are fit food for humans. Typical edible birds include chickens, turkeys, ducks, geese, pigeons, quail, ptarmigan and pheasants. In other words, what hunters call upland game birds and waterfowl. Most songbirds are also good for food. (Personally, I think I'd starve to death trying to eat the meat on a chickadee or wren!)

Forbidden birds and flying animals include all the birds of prey and the carrion eaters or scavengers. These include such things as bats, buzzards, crows, eagles, falcons, hawks, herons, jackdaws, kites, ostriches, owls, ravens, sea gulls, storks and vultures.

The only insects God approved for food are grasshoppers, locusts and crickets. All others are forbidden (Leviticus 11:20-23).

There you have it. This is God's list (not mine) of those animals, fish, birds and insects that are fit food for your body.

Chapter 4 Endnotes

1. Brennan, 1979. p. 93.
2. Brennan, 1979. p. 117.
3. Josephson, 1976. p. 112.
4. Josephson, 1976. p. 113.
5. Josephson, 1976. p. 113.
6. Your Word [Still] Is Truth, 1990.
7. Josephson, 1976. p. 107.
8. Josephson, 1976. p. 110.

Chapter 5

Results of Breaking God's Dietary Laws

Let's zero in now on some of the ways we harm our health by eating the flesh of these unclean animals.

Trichinosis

Many people still say to me, "Aha, God forbade eating pork because way back in those days people were ignorant of trichinosis. We now know how to kill these tiny worms so we don't have to worry."

They must think, "We're smarter than God!"

Is that so? A number of years ago, the surgeon-general of the United States estimated that 16 million people in the United States suffer from trichinosis.[1] Now who is laughing? Certainly not the 16 million infected people.

Trichinosis is hard to diagnose because its symptoms resemble many other diseases. Doctors have mis-diagnosed trichinosis as acute alcoholism, anemia, appendicitis, arthritis,[2] colitis, coughs, gall bladder troubles, heart disease, intestinal flu, lead poisoning, malaria, measles, meningitis, mumps, neuritis, peptic ulcers, poliomyelitis, ptomaine poisoning, rheumatism, scarlet fever, sinusitis, tuberculosis, typhoid fever and undulant fever.[3] In fact, doctors have incorrectly diagnosed trichinosis as approximately fifty different diseases.[4]

In a United States health report entitled, **The Complex Clinical Picture of Trichinosis and the Diagnosis of the Disease**, Dr. Maurice Hall reports that one study of cadavers from hospitals revealed "that out of 222 cases of trichinosis, **not one** was correctly diagnosed."[5]

This health report concludes that of "the total persons dying in the United States over the period of these surveys, one out of six was infected with the trichinae parasite [trichinella spiralis]."[6]

How about some sobering Canadian illustrations. In 1974, a **Wildlife Review** article revealed a grim picture of sickness and death to many of Canada's explorers in the past centuries.

In 1619-1620, a 64-man Danish expedition on the ship **Unicorn** was searching for the northwest passage. They wintered in the Churchill area of Hudson's Bay. There the men ate bear meat. Someone had told the cook, "just boil it slightly, and then keep it in vinegar for a night." By December, crew members were ailing. In June only three men remained alive. The captain's diary recorded, "the illness ... was very

Chapter 5: Results of Breaking God's Dietary Laws

peculiar and the sick were generally attacked by dysentery three weeks before they died." [7] These men died of trichinosis.

Here is another case. In 1897, a Swedish balloon expedition vanished in the Arctic. In 1930, explorers discovered the remains of this expedition, including some diaries. From these we now know that the men shot polar bears and ate the meat raw. Later, they developed stomach cramps, diarrhea, running noses, and severe fatigue. Dr. E. A. Tryde of Denmark noted these facts. He managed to obtain and examine meat scraps from a bear shot by the explorers. The meat scraps contained larvae of the worm responsible for trichinosis.[8] These explorers also died of trichinosis.

"Many other men have died under strange circumstances—mild weather and abundant food supplies. In light of what we now know of trichinosis, it seems very possible that their 'mysterious killer' has been found."[9]

Wildlife studies have shown that trichinosis is common in North American wildlife. It infects up to 50 percent of some species. All our meat-eating animals are susceptible.[10] Researchers have found trichinosis in bears, bobcats, cougars, coyotes, lynx, marten, skunks, weasels, and wolverines as well as several rodents.[11]

However, notice something staggering. Researchers have **never** found trichinosis in any animal species that God declared as fit food for humans! Why don't we ever learn?

Unfortunately, Evangelical Christians are the laughing stock of the world because they do not adhere to God's revealed dietary laws. However, among those people that do obey God's Word, such as Orthodox Jews and Seventh Day Adventists, there is an almost complete absence of trichinosis. Willard Wright and associates revealed this fact in a U.S. Health report. After much research they stated, "This survey amply demonstrates the protection afforded by adherence to the Mosaic Code."[12]

Even today we have not conquered trichinosis, not by any means. In fact, just detecting the trichinae larvae is a problem. Dr. Goldsborough tells us that in pork, the trichinae are often so minute and so nearly transparent that just finding them, even with a microscope, is indeed a difficult task, even for expert inspectors.[13] He also reports that when you see the words, 'U.S. Government Inspected and Passed,' those words do not mean that any official inspection whatever has been made for trichinosis. It has merely passed the routine inspection given all meats.[14]

Don't let anyone mislead you. Trichinosis is still a major problem today. In fact, as recently as March, 1991, trichinosis made the news again. This time the headlines read, "French ban American horse meat." This ban was imposed after 17 French people were admitted to hospitals with trichinosis after eating horse meat from a U.S. slaughterhouse.[15]

Trichinosis has no sure cure. There is no drug to kill the trichinae larvae. A laboratory in one northern U. S. university reported that "trichinae-laden swine flesh was heated to an unbelievably high temperature and then put under a microscope." Yet to the amazement of the technicians, some larvae were still alive and moving.[16]

However, trichinosis, bad as it is, is only one of many serious health problems that plague us because we eat these health-destroying forms of flesh.

Cancer

Not only are Seventh Day Adventists almost free from trichinosis, they are also relatively free from cancer.

Dr. Roland Phillips of Loma Linda University found "that the cancer death rate for Seventh Day Adventists in California is 50 to 70 per cent lower—depending upon the site—than the cancer death rate for the entire state."[17]

One reason God has blessed them with good health is that they generally keep His dietary laws concerning clean and unclean meats.

Furthermore, studies have implicated an excessive intake of animal fats and proteins as a cause of cancer.[18] These fats chemically break down into free radicals which damage cells[19] and can induce them to produce cancerous tumors.

"The fat story is real," declares Clifford Welsch, Michigan State University professor of pharmacology and toxicology. "There is overwhelming evidence in experimental animals that the amount and type of dietary fat markedly affects cancer." There seems to be a definite link between eating animal fat and the incidence of breast and colorectal cancer, and to a lesser extent, prostate, pancreatic and ovarian cancer.[20]

Elmer Josephson, who almost died of cancer himself before he started obeying God's dietary laws, tells of visiting a 70 year old lady. Cancer filled her body. Furthermore, she had numerous running sores. She asked him, "Why did God put this cancer on me? I have been a good, clean and moral woman."

He inquired as to the principal kind of meat she had eaten throughout the years. "Pork," she answered. "That was and still is our main meat dish."

He then asked her what her mother died of. "Cancer," she said.

"And what was her principal meat diet?" he asked her.

Again she answered, "Pork."[21]

Both of these ladies signed their own death warrants by disobeying God's dietary laws.

Rev. Josephson also tells of a friend of his who died of liver cancer. At one time his friend weighed about 250 pounds and loved pork chops. He would eat 6 or 7 at a meal. The last time he saw him before he died, his friend only "weighed about 80 pounds and his complexion was a deathly greenish yellow. He was upright, moral and godly—but he died."[22] He too, had disobeyed God's dietary laws. He too, had signed his own death warrant.

Did you know that modern Israel's parliament once passed a law banning raising, keeping or slaughtering any swine except in seven places that had large Christian populations?[23] Can you imagine that? The Christians, of all people, demanded the unclean diet! What a sad commentary on those who profess to believe the **whole** Bible.

Paralytic Shellfish Poisoning

Next to eating fat, pork and blood, probably more people in North America abuse God's dietary laws by eating shellfish—such as clams, crabs, lobsters, oysters, and prawns—than by eating any other unclean animal.

For example, the annual wholesale value of clams and oysters harvested along the coast of British Columbia in 1984 was $12,000,000.00. Total commercial shellfish sales in B. C. were 26 million dollars.[24] And that's just the commercial harvest. Think of the millions of pounds of shellfish taken privately in B. C. each year. Remember, these figures are just for British Columbia. Also think of the enormous shellfish harvests in the rest of the world.

Most people just don't think there is any harm in eating shellfish. In other words, they know better than God. Everything seems to be going well. Then comes the scare.

On July 11, 1986, federal fisheries officials banned the harvesting of clams, oysters and mussels along the entire British Columbia coast for the second time in six years.[25] Why? The dreaded red tide was back.

Red tide is the name given to a species of dinoflagellate or plankton[26] that periodically undergoes a massive population explosion. It then covers the surface of the sea with a red bloom. However, depending on which one of the 26 different organisms causes the problem,[27] it may appear pink, yellow, blue, green, orange, violet or brown.[28] These algae release a highly poisonous toxin into the water.

Now comes the insidious part. Most bivalve or hinged-shell shellfish including clams, oysters, mussels, scallops and cockles pick up the toxin laden algae because they are filter feeders. That is, they get both their food and oxygen by pumping prodigious quantities of water through their gills. For example, oysters filter about 4.5 liters of sea water each hour.[29]

As they filter the water, they concentrate many micro-organisms such as red tide toxins, chemicals, viruses and bacteria. Unlike fish, however, the shellfish are normally not affected by the poisons they ingest. They look all right. They act normal. However, they are deadly if eaten.

These shellfish become saturated with the poisons they have so efficiently filtered out of the water. Studies have shown that shellfish can contain 3 to 20 times the concentration of bacteria found in the water around them.[30]

These red tide toxins accumulate in the bodies of the shellfish in dangerous quantities. For example, the supposedly safe limit is less than 80 **micro**grams per 100 grams of meat. (A microgram is one millionth of a gram, a minute quantity indeed!) In B. C. in 1980, toxic levels reached 8,600 micrograms and one man died from eating such highly toxic butter clams. In 1986, B. C. authorities found toxic levels as high as a staggering 14,000 micrograms.[31] Now that's deadly!

Paralytic shellfish poisoning (PSP) is the most deadly algae-shellfish poisoning known.[32] How does the average person know whether the clams on his plate contain this deadly toxin? They usually find out when it is too late.

Chapter 5: Results of Breaking God's Dietary Laws

Paralytic shellfish poisoning symptoms typically appear from 20 minutes to two hours after eating toxic shellfish[33] although it may be much longer.

The paralytic shellfish poisoning toxin blocks the uptake of sodium in people. The nerves use a process called sodium exchange to pass messages throughout the body. With sodium blocked, symptoms such as numbness and tingling appear.[34] Victims feel this numbness and tingling on their lips, tongue, face, hands and feet. In severe cases they further experience nausea and vomiting[35] and ultimately death by suffocation when the nerves regulating breathing fail.[36]

And people do die. Each year around the world several hundred people die from paralytic shellfish poisoning.[37] Since ancient times, outbreaks of paralytic shellfish poisoning have appeared off both the East and West coasts of Canada, generally during the summer and fall.[38] In the few years before 1982, there were 182 cases of paralytic shellfish poisoning reported to Health and Welfare Canada. Three of them were fatal.[39]

Then too, fisheries officials are now finding red tide in formerly safe areas. For example, in October, 1988, South Puget Sound, the largest shellfish producing area in Washington State, was shut down for the first time because of a red tide outbreak.[40]

In June, 1990, an outbreak in Alaska killed one man and 13 others became ill after eating clams from Volcano Bay, near King Cove on the Alaskan Peninsula.[41]

Recent outbreaks in the Philippines and Guatemala killed more than 20 people in each location and put hundreds more in hospitals.[42]

In addition, scientists have discovered a generally non-fatal algae-related toxin called diarrhetic shellfish poisoning (DSP). They are now blaming it for the severe stomach upsets that people sometimes get after eating shellfish.[43]

There are many other toxins floating around in the ocean besides the one that causes paralytic shellfish poisoning. Scientists discover new ones from time to time. In December of 1987 (and again in October of 1988),[44] the newspapers were once more full of a new toxic scare. This time is was from people who had eaten mussels from Prince Edward Island. The mussels from Prince Edward Island were only rarely tested because "there had never been a paralytic shellfish poisoning in the entire history of the (province's) industry."[45] This time scientists did considerable research before they pinpointed this new toxin as domoic acid.[46]

Unfortunately, many people rejected God's warning about eating shellfish because they were just too wise in their own eyes. After all, what does God know about eating mussels? As a result, 150 people suffered.[47] Symptoms ranged from mild twitching and confusion to memory loss, stupor and coma.[48] Seventeen were hospitalized, several in intensive care,[49] and at least two died.[50]

Nor is that all. Of those that suffered, about one third have not fully recovered. One of the side effects of eating these tainted mussels is memory loss. Dr. Jeannie Teitelbaum of the Montreal Neurological Institute says some people have suffered such severe

Chapter 5: Results of Breaking God's Dietary Laws

memory loss they have had to be placed in nursing homes.[51] Those less severely affected now have to rely on their calendars, agendas and notes they make for themselves so they know what to do next.[52]

Paralytic shellfish poisoning comes from one species of plankton while domoic acid is a byproduct of a type of seaweed. How many other toxins have yet to be discovered? How many more people will die before man begins to heed God's dietary laws?

In 1990, Dr. Ron Guiderian studied a disease, called paragonimiasis, that infects the lungs of people and mimics the symptoms of tuberculosis. Paragonimiasis is found in Latin America. So far, Eucador seems to have the highest infection rate. "This disease is transmitted to humans only when they eat certain species of infected fresh-water crabs, a favorite food among people who live along rivers in Eucador's tropical and sub-tropical regions." So far more than 2,000 cases have been reported.[53]

Contaminated shellfish can take months to clean the toxins out of their systems.[54] Some never do. Nor is cooking really the answer. Cooking normally kills any bacteria found in shellfish, but it has little or no effect on the paralytic shellfish poisoning toxin.[55]

Make no mistake about it. Shellfish are not fit food for humans. Like pigs, they are garbage eaters. "Sewage makes clams grow bigger and faster" according to fisheries officer, Bob Tupniak. That's why so many people dig for them in such places.[56]

Imagine, trying to keep healthy, yet swallowing animals that suck up sewage, toxins and bacteria for a living. A person would have to be nuts to do that. If you want seafood, eat fish since they are not normally affected by these various toxins.[57] They are the seafood that God wanted you to eat anyway.

Liver Cirrhosis

A recent report by Dr. Amin Nanji, Head of Clinical Biochemistry at the Ottawa General Hospital reveals that in Canada the death rate from liver cirrhosis is directly related—now hold your hat—not to alcohol consumption, but to **pork** consumption.[58] However, alcohol and pork combined launch a devastating attack on the liver. When your liver dies, you die. Why trifle with either of these so-called foods?

Chapter 5 Endnotes

1 Robinson, 1954. p. 5.
2 Josephson, 1976. p. 59.
3 Robinson, 1954. pp. 7-8.
4 Josephson, 1976. p. 59.
5 Robinson, 1954. p. 7.
6 Robinson, 1954. p. 8.
7 Friis, 1974. p. 14.
8 Friis, 1974. pp. 14-15.
9 Friis, 1974. p. 15.
10 Friis, 1974. p. 15.
11 Friis, 1974. p. 15.
12 Robinson, 1954. p. 8.
13 Josephson, 1976. p. 58.
14 Josephson, 1976. pp. 58-59.
15 French Ban American Horse Meat, 1991. p. A16.
16 Josephson, 1976. p. 59.
17 Mormons' Faith Pays Off...in Fewer Cancer Cases, 1975.
18 Tait, 1984.
19 Carcinogens Common in Diets, 1983.
20 Your Word [Still] Is Truth, 1990.
21 Josephson, 1976. pp. 73-74.

Chapter 5: Results of Breaking God's Dietary Laws

22 Josephson, 1976. p. 75.
23 Josephson, 1976. p. 52.
24 Pynn, July 11, 1986. p. A1.
25 Pynn, July 11, 1986. p. A1.
26 Beltrame, 1987. p. A3.
27 Beltrame, 1987. p. A3.
28 Strauss, 1987. pp. D1, D6.
29 Strauss, 1987. pp. D1, D6.
30 Strauss, 1987. pp. D1, D6.
31 Pynn, July 17, 1986. p. A1.
32 Strauss, 1987. pp. D1, D6.
33 Pynn, July 11, 1986. p. A1.
34 Strauss, 1987. pp. D1, D6.
35 Pynn, July 17, 1986. p. A1.
36 Strauss, 1987. pp. D1, D6.
37 Strauss, 1987. pp. D1, D6.
38 Strauss, 1987. pp. D1, D6.
39 Strauss, 1987. pp. D1, D6.
40 Red Tide Strikes Puget Sound, 1988. p. A16.
41 Shellfish Toxin Hits Alaskans, 1990.
42 Strauss, 1987. pp. D1, D6.
43 Strauss, 1987. pp. D1, D6.
44 Shellfish Toxin Found in PEI, 1988.
45 Beltrame, 1987. p. A3.
46 Mussel Toxin Pinpointed by Scientists, 1987. p. A1.
47 Mussel Victims Losing Memories, 1989.
48 Mussel Toxin Cure in Sight, 1988.
49 Health Officials Hope Worst Is Over, 1987. p. B10.
50 Mussel Toxin Cure in Sight, 1988.
51 Mussel Victims Losing Memories, 1989.
52 Mussel Victims Losing Memories, 1989.
53 HCJB Tests Drug for TB-like Disease, 1990. p. 12.
54 Strauss, 1987. pp. D1, D6.
55 Strauss, 1987. pp. D1, D6.
56 Red-Tide Worries Not a Shell Game, 1986. p. A10.
57 Pynn, July 11, 1986. p. A1.
58 Hoskins, 1986. p. 32.

Chapter 6

Unclean Animals Aptly Named

In the Bible, God calls all animals unclean that are not fit food for humans. Nor is this just a euphemism. Such animals are indeed the scavengers and garbage collectors of the earth. How unclean animals process this food (garbage) in their stomachs, compared to the clean animals, is revealing.

The clean animals, those that chew the cud and divide the hoof such as sheep, goats and cattle, have three stomachs. They use these stomachs for purifying their food of all poisonous and harmful matter. It takes them over twenty-four hours to turn their clean vegetable food into flesh. Their flesh is clean, not merely ceremonially clean, but hygienically and physiologically clean and wholesome for humans.[1]

In comparison, pigs, for example, have much more primitive stomachs and limited excretory organs. It only takes four hours after a pig has eaten his polluted, putrid swill until a man may eat the same second hand off the ribs of the pig.[2]

God condemns pork as unclean because by its very nature it is poisonous, diseased and deadly. Eating pork is a prime cause of much of our poor health. It causes such things as blood diseases, weak stomachs, liver troubles, eczema, consumption, tumors and cancer.[3]

Dr. J. H. Kellog, in a study called **The Scientific View of the Hog** shows that the hog is a dangerous carrier of disease because the animal is diseased itself.

Dr. Kellog pointed out that the fat on the pig is not healthy fat, but results from the pig's inability to throw off its impurities. "Consequently," says Dr. Kellog, "this flood of disease is crowded out of the veins and arteries into the tissues, and so, is accumulated as fat. Lard then, is nothing more than extract of a diseased carcass."[4]

I could go on and on telling about other unclean animals like the dog and the dog-fish shark, both of which have livers so high in vitamin A that eating them is fatal to man. This is in sharp contrast to the nutritious livers of the clean animals such as cattle. However, there is no need for more examples. You get the picture. God didn't make any mistakes. Whether we know the scientific or medical reasons why the meat of certain animals is bad for us or not doesn't matter. We must obey God for He has our physical well-being in mind.

Why not heed God's Word and live? "Do not be deceived, God is not mocked; for whatever a man sows, that he will also reap" (Galatians 6:7).

Therefore, God reminds us once again, "You shall therefore distinguish between clean animals and unclean, between unclean birds and clean, and you shall not make yourselves abominable [or loathsome] by beast or by bird, or by any kind of living thing that creeps on the ground, **which I have separated from you as unclean** [or defiled]. And you shall be holy to Me," (Leviticus 20:25-26). How could God make Himself any clearer?

Chapter 6 Endnotes

1   Josephson, 1976. p. 46.
2   Josephson, 1976. p. 46.
3   Josephson, 1976. p. 47.
4   Robinson, 1954. p. 9.

Chapter 7

But the New Testament Says . . .

This chapter is vitally important. Most Christians ignorantly assert, "There are many New Testament passages that supersede those Old Testament dietary laws." Is that so? Let's look at some of those passages and discover what they really teach.

The most often quoted passage in favor of eating all kinds of filthy flesh is the story of Peter's vision. In this episode, Peter saw an enormous sheet let down from heaven containing all manner of unclean animals. Furthermore, he heard a voice from heaven saying, "'Rise, Peter, kill and eat.'

But Peter said, 'Not so, Lord! For **I have never eaten anything common or unclean**.'

And a voice spoke to him again the second time, 'What God has cleansed [declared clean] you must not call common.'" (Acts 10:13-15).

Now notice two specific points in this passage. First, Peter declared that he **never** ate unclean animals. Second, in verse 17, Peter "wondered [was

Keep Yourself Healthy

perplexed] within himself what this vision which he had seen meant." Peter didn't understand what God was telling him. In the Old Testament, God had said not to eat unclean animals. Now God was apparently telling him the opposite. Yet Peter also knew that God had said, "I am the Lord, **I do not change**" (Malachi 3:6). No wonder this vision puzzled him.

God, however, did not keep Peter in the dark for long. In Acts 10:28 we read, "Then he [Peter] said to them, 'You know how unlawful it is for a Jewish man to keep company with or go to one of another nation. But God has shown me that I should not call any **man** common or unclean." God was not talking about food at all. He was talking about taking the gospel message to the nations of the world! Too often, people don't read to the end of this story to find out its true meaning.

In another passage beginning at Matthew 15:10 (and its parallel passage in Mark 7:15), Jesus said, "Hear and understand: Not what goes into the mouth defiles a man: but what comes out of the mouth, this defiles a man."

Is this passage talking about eating unclean animals? Of course not! Why not? First, Jesus was talking about food in general, not just unclean meats. Second, the Pharisees to whom Jesus was speaking kept the **letter of the law** as regards eating unclean foods. They wouldn't even dream of eating pork!

So what was the problem? The Pharisees said that if you didn't wash your hands before you touched your food, you were unclean. Notice that Jesus declared plainly, "These are the things [see verse 19] which defile a man, but **to eat with unwashed hands**

Chapter 7: But the New Testament Says...

does not defile a man" (Matthew 15:20). Again we need to read right through to the end of the passage to get its full meaning. Only then can we "rightly divide the word of truth" (II Timothy 2:15).

This next passage has led far too many Christians astray because they didn't understand what God said. It reads: "Now the Spirit expressly says that in latter times some will depart from the faith, giving heed to deceiving spirits and doctrines of demons, speaking lies in hypocrisy, having their own conscience seared with a hot iron, forbidding to marry, and commanding to abstain from foods which God created to be received with thanksgiving by those who believe and know the truth. For every creature of God is good and nothing is to be refused if it is received with thanksgiving; for it is sanctified by the word of God and prayer" (I Timothy 4:1-5).

These verses seem straightforward. Obviously, you can eat all kinds of meats as long as you are thankful and say grace before eating them. Right?

Again, nothing could be further from the truth! So what is the truth?

First, this passage is for the latter times—that is, for us today. Now notice, some **leave the truth** and listen (the Greek says adhere to) evil lying spirits. What is the result? They lie, their conscience is branded with the mark of the devil and they start promoting some **new** doctrines that God did not give.

The first false doctrine they propounded was "forbidding to marry." What so-called Christian church forbids its priests to marry? Is this scriptural? No, it is not. It is a lie from the devil himself.

The second false doctrine perpetrated was in commanding to abstain from foods (the Greek word does not limit itself to meats) which God created to be received with thanksgiving. Again, up until a few years ago, what so-called Christian church forbad eating meat, even clean meat, on Fridays? Only fish could be eaten. Remember the fish Fridays? Was this from God? Of course not. Obviously, then, it came from the devil also.

Nowhere did God forbid us from eating a roast of beef on Friday, or any other day of the week for that matter. This is what this verse is talking about. Not whether an animal was good for food or not. Fortunately, evangelical Christians rejected the fish-only business on Fridays.

Only clean animals are referred to here in the first place. How do we know? Notice the clause, "which God created **to be received**" (verse 3). The truth is that God created certain animals to be received as food for humans and certain animals to be rejected as scavengers and unfit for human consumption. This is further emphasized, "by those who believe and know the truth." What truth? In this case, God is referring to the truth as found in the Old Testament's dietary laws.

So far so good. Now in verse 4 there seems to be a problem. "For every creature **of God** is good and nothing is to be refused." What is this verse really saying, especially in light of the above verses? Particularly notice the phrase, "of God." Why is it here? Why doesn't this verse just read, "every creature is good?" After all, didn't God create all creatures? Of course He did. God added this extra phrase to **limit** the meaning of this verse to the **clean** animals. How do we know that? The next verse explains, "For it is

Chapter 7: But the New Testament Says...

sanctified [or set apart] by the word of God." The Word of God is the Bible. Now, in relation to animals and food, what was sanctified or set apart in the Bible? This obviously refers to the passage in Leviticus 11 where God set apart the clean animals for human consumption.

Therefore, this passage does not give us license to eat anything we choose. Instead, it refers us back to the Old Testament dietary laws for our authority.

If you disagree, consider the alternative. If every creature is good, then this would include every poisonous reptile, venomous serpent and deadly viper. It would include the wriggling mass of loathsome maggots and worms that feed on dead rotten carcasses. It would even include cannibalism.[1]

If you still feel this is the correct interpretation, how about trying this sumptuous dinner? Pit viper cocktail; your choice of thunder lizard or bush mouse soup, round-worm/termite salad, and juicy rare rat roast. If you want something lighter, try a cockroach, or black widow spider sandwich. If you love steak, you have a choice of dog, sloth, or tomcat. For dessert, how about maggot cake and a delicious creepy-crawly sundae?

Is this what you really want? You had better start eating it if **every creature** is good for dietary purposes.

Praying over this mess of filth can't make it any better, can it? Of course not! God does not honor you while you break His dietary laws.

Perhaps a parallel illustration will make this clear. For example, suppose you pray over a person,

49

then kill him. Does praying over him make killing him all right even though you know that God explicitly commands, "You shall not murder" (Exodus 20:13)? Of course not. Therefore, if you can't justify breaking one of God's moral laws, how can you justify breaking one of God's dietary laws? After all, God made both.

Another New Testament problem passage reads, "I know and am convinced by the Lord Jesus that there is nothing unclean of itself; but to him who considers anything to be unclean, to him it is unclean" (Romans 14:14). Does this verse mean if you think it is all right to eat pork, it is okay for you? However, if I think it is wrong, then I cannot eat pork? Not at all. This passage is not talking about clean and unclean animals, but is contrasting vegetarians to meat eaters. Take it in context. In verses 1 and 2 notice what Paul said, "Receive one who is **weak in the faith**, but not to disputes over doubtful things. For one believes he may eat all things [that is, both meat and vegetables], but he who is weak eats only vegetables [that is, a vegetarian]." Problem resolved.

No doubt there are many other New Testament passages that could give problems to the unwary. However, when we examine these passages carefully, we do not find any real conflict with the Old Testament dietary laws.

Now let's look at a New Testament passage that commands us to keep the Old Testament dietary laws. Yes, there really are some. How is this for an unlikely passage? "As He [God] who called you is holy, you also be holy in all your conduct, because it is written, 'Be holy, for I am holy'" (I Peter 1:15-16).

From which book was this quote by Peter taken? Surprise, Leviticus chapter 11, the very chapter

Chapter 7: But the New Testament Says...

where God gives us the dietary laws in the first place! Therefore, part of being holy in all our conduct **includes abstaining from eating unclean animals**.

Paul also admonishes us, "I beseech you therefore, brethren, by the mercies of God, that you present **your bodies a living sacrifice**, **holy**, **acceptable to God**, which is your **reasonable** service" (Romans 12:1).

Now consider this. **All** sacrificial animals were clean animals such as cattle, sheep and goats. They were **never** unclean animals such as pigs, horses and rabbits. This is because all sacrifices had to be holy (clean and pure) in order to be acceptable to God.

If we eat unclean animals, we defile our bodies. God declared, "If anyone defiles the temple of God, **God will destroy him**, For the temple of God is **holy**, **which temple you are**" (1 Corinthians 3:17). Perhaps we should start looking at our bodies (temples of God) from God's point of view. If we don't, God judges us with disease, sickness and death.

God declares, "I have stretched out My hands all day long to a **rebellious people**, who walk in a way that is **not good**, according to **their own thoughts**; A people who **provoke me to anger continually** to My face" (Isaiah 65:2-3). Why? "Who eat **swine's flesh**, and the **broth of abominable things [unclean meats]** is in their vessels; Who say, 'Keep to yourself, do not come near me, for **I am holier than you**'" (Isaiah 65:4-5)!

This description fits far too many Christians who are proud they can eat any unclean animal they want, no matter what God says. Would you want to be in their shoes when God promises, "Those who ... eat swine's flesh and the abomination and the mouse, **shall be consumed** together," says the Lord (Isaiah 66:17).

Did the Christians in the New Testament continue to follow the Old Testament dietary laws? Let's look at two of the most famous men in the New Testament and see.

The apostle Paul, the greatest missionary of all time, tells us, "But this I confess to you, that according to the Way which they call a sect, so I worship the God of my fathers, **believing all things which are written in the law** and in the Prophets" (Acts 24:14).

Paul was living in New Testament times. Did he keep the Old Testament dietary laws? You bet he did! He believed and thus kept God's laws as written in the Torah. The Torah comprises the first five books of the Bible, which include both passages on the dietary laws.

How about the Lord Jesus Himself? Did He keep the Old Testament dietary laws? In the New Testament, there is not even a hint that Jesus ever violated the Old Testament dietary laws. There is absolutely no evidence that He ever ate any unclean animal. If He had, He could not have stood before the crowd and challenged, "Which of you convicts Me of [any] sin" (John 8:46)?

Jesus was sinless. Therefore, He faithfully obeyed God's laws, including God's dietary laws for good health. Can we do less than to follow the Lord's example?

Solomon, the wisest man that ever lived, near the end of his life concluded, "Fear God, and **keep**

Chapter 7: But the New Testament Says...

His commandments: for this is the **whole duty** of man" (Ecclesiastes 12:13, KJV).

God is a loving and merciful God. Therefore, let's keep His dietary laws. Then, "whatever we ask we receive from Him [including good health], because we **keep His commandments** and **do those things that are pleasing in His sight**" (I John 3:22). Could we ask for more? Remember, God wants us to be healthy!

Chapter 7 Endnotes

1   Josephson, 1976. p. 88.

Literature Cited

Beltrame, Julian. Mysterious Shellfish Poison Difficult to Find or Prevent In: *Calgary Herald*. Calgary, Alberta. December 15, 1987.

Brennan, Dr. Richard O. 1979. *Coronary? Cancer? God's Answer: Prevent It*. Harvest House Publishers. Irvine, California, 92714.

Carcinogens common in diets. In: *Calgary Herald*. Calgary, Alberta. September 21, 1983.

Friis, Laura. 1974. Trichinosis, Was This the Arctic Killer? In: *Wildlife Review*. Summer, 1974. Victoria, B.C.

French Ban American Horse Meat. In: *Calgary Herald*. Calgary, Alberta. March 21, 1991.

HCJB Tests Drug for TB-like Disease In: *Around The World*. World Radio Missionary Fellowship. Miami, Florida. Summer, 1990.

Health Officials Hope Worst Is Over. In: *Calgary Herald*. Calgary, Alberta. December 10, 1987.

Hoskins, Carolyn. Pork Linked to Liver Cirrhosis. In: *Canadian Science News*. Reprinted in Identity Magazine. January, 1986.

Josephson, Elmer A. 1976. *God's Key to Health and Happiness*. Fleming H. Revell Company. Old Tappen, New Jersey.

Leprosy. In: *Encyclopaedia Britannica*. 1910. (Eleventh Edition). Cambridge University Press. London. Vol. 16

Leprosy. In: *World Book Encyclopedia*. 1979. WorldBook-Child-Craft International, Inc. Chicago, Illinois, 60654. Vol 12.

McMillen, S. I. 1978. *None of These Diseases*. Fleming H. Revell Company. Old Tappen, New Jersey.

Mormons' Faith Pays Off... in Fewer Cancer Cases. In: *Victoria Times*. Victoria, B.C. March 29, 1975.

Mussel Toxin Cure in Sight. In: *Calgary Herald*. Calgary, Alberta. October 31, 1988.

Mussel Toxin Pinpointed by Scientists. In: *Calgary Herald*. Calgary, Alberta. December 19, 1987.

Mussel Victims Losing Memories. In: *Calgary Herald*. Calgary, Alberta. January 7, 1989.

Pynn, Larry. Red Tide Warning Hits Most of B.C. In: *Vancouver Sun*. Vancouver, B.C. July 11, 1986.

Pynn, Larry. Red-Tide Toxins Reach Deadly Level. In: *Vancouver Sun*. Vancouver, B.C. July 17, 1986.

Red Tide Strikes Puget Sound. In: *The Vancouver Sun*. Vancouver, British Columbia. October 11, 1988.

Red-Tide Worries Not a Shell Game. In: *Vancouver Sun*. Vancouver, B.C. July 17, 1986.

Robinson, Herbert. 1954. *Suicide Through Eating.* Mimeographed Manuscript. Covenant Tabernacle. Vancouver, B.C.

Shellfish Toxin Found in PEI. In: *The Globe and Mail.* October 24, 1988.

Shellfish Toxin Hits Alaskans. In: *Calgary Herald.* Calgary, Alberta. June 27, 1990.

Spanish-American War. In: *Encyclopaedia Britannica.* 1910. Vol. 25.

Strauss, Stephen. "An Ancient and Deadly Phenomenon." In: *The Globe and Mail.* December 19, 1987.

Tait, Mark. Clean Living Helps to Stave Off Cancer. In: *Calgary Herald.* Calgary, Alberta. March 30, 1984.

Your Word [Still] Is Truth. In: *The Plain Truth.* February, 1991. Reprinted from the Los Angeles Times, June 26, 1990.

Bible-Based Books by the Same Author

Integrity First Books in the series:

Get More (Much More) Out of Your Bible

by Neil G. Bauman, Ph.D.

If you have enjoyed this book and would like to learn more about the deeper things in God's Word, you may be interested in some of the other books by Dr. Neil. Each book is packed with the "hidden manna" from God's Word. You can obtain these books from www.integrityfirstpublications.com.

The Real Christmas Story—The Truth About the Events Surrounding Jesus' Birth ($26.99)

Christmas is overgrown with so many "warm fuzzy" traditions that few people know the truth about the real Christmas story anymore. If you sincerely want to know the true Christmas story this book is for you. However, be prepared to be shocked, surprised, thrilled (and perhaps even grossed out at times) by what you will discover. It will change the way you view Christmas forever. You will learn the true day of Jesus' birth, the thrilling story of who Mary really was, the "secret sign" of the swaddling clothes, the mysterious star of Bethlehem revealed at last, the amazing story of the Magi and much more. (356 pages).

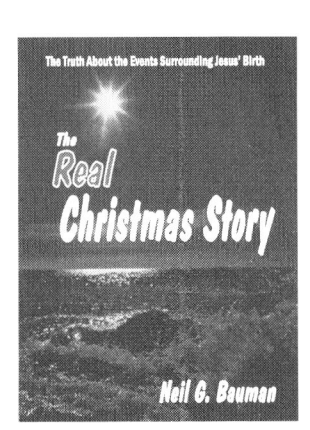

Keep Yourself Healthy—God's Principles of Good Health ($12.95)

God loves us and wants us to be healthy! Yet far too many people are sick because they either don't know or deliberately ignore God's instructions for good health. **Keep Yourself Healthy** is a brief introduction to some of God's rules for good health. Many Christians falsely believe that because we live under grace, not under the law, we do not have to keep God's food rules for good health. This book exposes this myth for what it really is—a lie to keep us from enjoying God's vibrant health. You owe it to yourself to read this book and then consider if your poor health is the result of flaunting God's principles of good health. (60 pages).

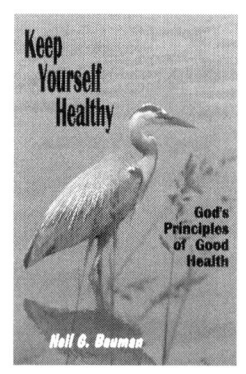

You can order the foregoing books from the
Integrity First Publications
web site at
http://www.integrityfirstpublications.com
or order them from the address below

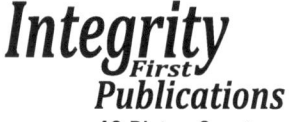

Integrity First Publications
49 Piston Court,
Stewartstown, PA 17363-8322
Phone: (717) 993-8555
FAX: (717) 993-6661
Email: info@IntegrityFirstPublications.com
Website: http://www.IntegrityFirstPublications.com

Made in the USA
Charleston, SC
19 October 2011